5-MUNITE CORE EXERCISE FOR SENIORS OVER 60

A Senior's Guide to Stronger Cores and Active Living

Jimmy Ledet

Table of Contents

INTRODUCTION

Welcome to "5-Minute Core Exercises for Seniors Over 60"! First off, let's have a virtual high-five for taking this exciting step towards strengthening your core and embracing a healthier, more vibrant you. Whether you're flipping through these pages with a gleeful grin or a curious brow, know that you're not alone on this journey. Picture me, your friendly guide, cheering you on with pom-poms in hand (metaphorically, of course).

Now, before we dive headfirst into the world of core exercises, let's have a heart-to-heart. I get it. The idea of exercising, especially as we gracefully age like fine wine (or cheese, whichever you prefer), can feel daunting. Maybe the thought of crunches and planks makes you roll your eyes faster than a teenager texting. Or perhaps you've had a love-hate relationship with fitness since your aerobics days in neon spandex.

Guess what? You're not alone in those sentiments. We're in this together, navigating the twists and turns of maintaining our health and vitality as we venture through the golden years. So, consider me your trusty companion, here to sprinkle some empathy, understanding, and maybe even a dash of humor into our fitness escapades.

Let's address the elephant in the room (or should I say, the "senior" in the room?): core exercises. Ah, the core. It's like the Swiss Army knife of our bodies, responsible for everything from standing tall like a redwood tree to effortlessly reaching for that top shelf cookie jar. Yet, let's be real, giving our core the attention it deserves isn't always at the top of our to-do list.

But fear not, my seasoned friend! This book isn't about grueling hours at the gym or pushing yourself to extremes. Nope, we're all about efficiency here. Five minutes. That's all it takes. Think about it: that's less time than it takes to microwave popcorn or scroll through your grandkids' latest Instagram posts. And hey, if you want to multitask while doing these exercises, I won't judge. Just don't blame me if you accidentally fling your smartphone across the room during a particularly intense plank.

So, why should you care about your core? Well, besides the fact that it's like the sturdy foundation of a house, keeping everything else in place, having a strong core can seriously level up your quality of life. Picture this: you're strolling through the park with your friends, regaling them with tales of your glory days, and suddenly, you trip on a rogue acorn (those sneaky little things). Instead of face-planting into the grass like a rookie, your strong core kicks in, keeping you upright and saving you from embarrassment. See? Core strength is the real MVP.

But I get it. You might be thinking, "Sure, core exercises sound great, but where do I even begin? And can I do them without feeling like a contortionist in Cirque du Soleil?" Fear not, my friend. We're going to start slow, keep things simple, and most importantly, have fun along the way. No need for fancy equipment or bending yourself into pretzel-like shapes. Just you, me, and a willingness to give your core the love and attention it deserves.

Throughout this book, you'll find everything you need to embark on your 5-minute core exercise journey. From understanding the basics of core fitness to practical tips for staying motivated, consider this your roadmap to a stronger, more resilient core. And hey, if you stumble along the way (figuratively, not literally), that's okay. We'll dust ourselves off, share a laugh, and keep moving forward together.

So, dear reader, are you ready to embark on this adventure with me? Let's flip the page, lace up our imaginary sneakers, and dive into the wonderful world of 5-minute core exercises for seniors over 60. Trust me, your core will thank you, and who knows, you might even discover a newfound love for those crunches and planks. Okay, maybe "love" is pushing it, but hey, stranger things have happened.

Here's to stronger cores, brighter smiles, and countless "I told you so" moments when you impress your friends with your newfound strength. Let's do this!

Warmest regards,

UNDERSTANDING CORE FITNESS

What is the Core?

When we talk about the core, we're not just referring to those six-pack abs you see plastered on fitness magazines or the elusive quest for a beach-ready body. No, the core is so much more than that. Think of it as the central powerhouse of your body, akin to the engine of a car or the foundation of a skyscraper. It's where all movement originates and where stability and balance are cultivated.

So, what exactly makes up this powerhouse we call the core? Well, it's not just about those superficial abdominal muscles (although they do play a part). The core actually comprises a complex network of muscles that span from your pelvis to your shoulders and everything in between. We're talking about muscles like the transverse abdominis, internal and external oblique's, rectus abdominis, erector spinae, and the multifidus, just to name a few.

But here's the kicker: the core isn't just about what you see on the surface. Sure, having a toned midsection is nice, but true core strength goes much deeper (pun intended). It's about cultivating stability and strength from the inside out, creating a solid foundation that supports you in all your daily activities, whether it's bending down to tie your shoes or reaching for that top shelf in the pantry.

Now, you might be wondering, "But why should I care about my core?" Ah, my friend, that's where things get interesting.

Importance of Core Strength for Seniors

Let's face it: as we gracefully age (emphasis on the graceful part), maintaining our strength and mobility becomes increasingly important. Gone are the days of effortlessly hoisting heavy boxes or springing out of bed with the energy of a caffeinated squirrel. But fear not, my seasoned friend, because that's where core strength swoops in to save the day.

You see, as we age, our bodies naturally undergo changes. Muscle mass decreases, joints become stiffer, and balance can become a bit wobbly (quite literally). That's where a strong core comes into play. By nurturing and strengthening those deep core muscles, we can mitigate the effects of aging, helping us maintain stability, mobility, and independence well into our golden years.

But the benefits of core strength go beyond just physical prowess. Oh no, we're talking about a whole-body transformation here. When your core is strong and stable, you'll notice improvements in posture, reducing the likelihood of pesky aches and pains that often plague us as we age. Plus, a strong core can enhance your balance and coordination, reducing the risk of falls and keeping you steady on your feet.

But perhaps most importantly, cultivating core strength can boost your overall quality of life. Whether it's playing with your grandkids, gardening in the backyard, or simply going for a leisurely stroll, having a strong core means you can tackle life's adventures with confidence and vitality. And let's be honest, who doesn't want to feel like a superhero, ready to take on whatever challenges come their way?

Common Core Strength Myths Debunked

Ah, myths. They're like those stubborn weeds in your garden that just won't go away, no matter how many times you try to pull them out. When it comes to core strength, there's no shortage of myths and misconceptions floating around. But fear not, my friend, because I'm here to set the record straight and debunk some of the most common myths about core fitness.

- **Myth #1:** Crunches are the key to a strong core. Ah, the humble crunch. It's been the go-to exercise for core enthusiasts for decades. But here's the truth: while crunches can certainly help strengthen the superficial abdominal muscles, they're not the be-all and end-all of core training. In fact, focusing solely on crunches can neglect other important muscles in the core, leading to imbalances and potential injury. Instead, opt for a well-rounded approach that targets all aspects of core strength, including stability, flexibility, and endurance.

- **Myth #2:** Core exercises are only for young, fit people. Wrong! Core exercises are for everyone, regardless of age or fitness level. In fact, they're especially important for seniors, who may be more prone to issues like poor posture, back pain, and decreased mobility. The key is to start slow, listen to your body, and gradually progress as you build strength and confidence. Remember, it's never too late to reap the benefits of a strong core, no matter how many candles are on your birthday cake.

- **Myth #3:** You need fancy equipment to strengthen your core. Sure, having access to fancy gym equipment can be nice, but it's certainly not necessary for building a strong core. In fact, some of the most effective core exercises can be done with nothing more than your own body weight. Think planks, bridges, and bird dogs, just to name a few. And if you do want to add some resistance to your workouts, you can easily do so with simple tools like resistance bands or light dumbbells. So, no excuses – get ready to strengthen that core, no fancy equipment required. Understanding core fitness is about more than just doing a few sit-ups or holding a plank for a minute. It's about cultivating strength, stability, and resilience from the inside out, empowering you to live life to the fullest, no matter your age or fitness level. So, let's banish those myths, embrace the power of our core, and embark on this journey together towards a stronger, healthier you.

ADVANTAGES OF 5-MINUTE CORE EXERCISES

In today's fast-paced world, finding time for exercise can be challenging. Between work, family commitments, and other responsibilities, many individuals struggle to prioritize physical activity. However, incorporating 5-minute core exercises into your daily routine offers numerous advantages, making it easier to maintain a strong and healthy core despite a busy schedule. In this chapter, we'll explore the advantages of 5-minute core exercises, including their time-efficiency, accessibility, and role in establishing a sustainable exercise habit.

Time-Efficiency: Maximizing Results in Minimal Time

One of the most significant advantages of 5-minute core exercises is their time-efficiency. In just a few minutes a day, you can effectively target and strengthen your core muscles, leading to improved stability, balance, and overall fitness. Unlike traditional workout routines that may require 30 minutes or more, 5-minute core exercises allow you to maximize results in minimal time, making them ideal for busy individuals who struggle to find time for longer workouts.

The key to the time-efficiency of 5-minute core exercises lies in their focus on high-intensity, targeted movements. By selecting exercises that engage multiple muscle groups simultaneously and incorporating interval training principles, you can create short yet effective workouts that provide significant benefits in a fraction of the time. For example, exercises like planks, mountain climbers, and bicycle crunches can effectively engage the core muscles while also elevating heart rate and promoting calorie burn.

Additionally, the short duration of 5-minute core exercises makes them easy to fit into even the busiest of schedules. Whether you have a few minutes before work, during your lunch break, or before bed, there's always time to squeeze in a quick core workout. By breaking down barriers to exercise and eliminating the need for extended time commitments, 5-minute core exercises empower individuals to prioritize their health and well-being, no matter how hectic their schedule may be.

Accessibility: Incorporating Core Workouts into Busy Schedules

Another advantage of 5-minute core exercises is their accessibility. Unlike traditional gym workouts that may require specialized equipment or a dedicated exercise space, 5-minute core exercises can be performed virtually anywhere, with minimal equipment or space requirements. This accessibility makes it easy to incorporate core workouts into your daily routine, whether you're at home, in the office, or traveling.

Many 5-minute core exercises require nothing more than your body weight, making them perfect for at-home workouts or when you're on the go. Exercises like planks, bridges, and Russian twists can be performed in the comfort of your living room, bedroom, or even in a hotel room while traveling. Additionally, minimal equipment such as a yoga mat or stability ball can further enhance the effectiveness and variety of your 5-minute core workouts.

The accessibility of 5-minute core exercises also removes common barriers to exercise, such as cost, time, and convenience. Unlike gym memberships or fitness classes, which may require financial investment and travel time, 5-minute core exercises are free and can be done anytime, anywhere. This accessibility makes it easier for individuals of all fitness levels and backgrounds to prioritize their core health and incorporate regular exercise into their daily lives.

Consistency: Establishing a Sustainable Exercise Habit

Consistency is key to achieving and maintaining a strong and healthy core. However, for many individuals, maintaining consistency with exercise can be challenging, especially when faced with busy schedules and competing priorities. The beauty of 5-minute core exercises lies in their ability to facilitate consistency by making exercise more manageable, accessible, and enjoyable.

By breaking down exercise into manageable 5-minute sessions, individuals can establish a sustainable exercise habit that fits seamlessly into their daily routine. Instead of feeling overwhelmed by the prospect of hour-long workouts, individuals can approach exercise as a series of small, achievable goals that add up over time. This approach not only reduces feelings of intimidation and fatigue but also fosters a sense of accomplishment and motivation to continue.

Additionally, the accessibility of 5-minute core exercises makes it easier to maintain consistency, even on the busiest of days. Rather than skipping workouts altogether due to time constraints or lack of access to a gym, individuals can perform quick core exercises wherever they are, ensuring that they stay on track with their fitness goals. Over time, this consistency builds momentum, leading to lasting changes in behavior and overall health.

Furthermore, the regular practice of 5-minute core exercises can lead to tangible improvements in core strength, stability, and overall fitness, further reinforcing the importance of consistency. As individuals begin to experience the benefits of their efforts, such as improved posture, reduced lower back pain, and increased energy levels, they're motivated to continue their exercise routine and prioritize their core health.

5-minute core exercises offer numerous advantages, including time-efficiency, accessibility, and the ability to establish a sustainable exercise habit. By incorporating quick core workouts into your daily routine, you can maximize results in minimal time, regardless of how busy your schedule may be. Whether you're at home, in the office, or on the go, there's always time to prioritize your core health and well-being. With consistency, dedication, and the right mindset, you can achieve a strong, resilient core and enjoy the many benefits of regular exercise.

DISADVANTAGES OF 5-MINUTE CORE EXERCISES

In our quest for efficiency and convenience, it's easy to overlook potential drawbacks. While 5-minute core exercises offer undeniable benefits, it's essential to acknowledge their limitations and address potential disadvantages. In this chapter, we'll explore the disadvantages of 5-minute core exercises, including challenges in achieving high-intensity workouts, the potential for plateaus, and the need to tailor exercises to individual fitness levels.

Limited Intensity: Challenges in Achieving High-Intensity Workouts

One of the primary disadvantages of 5-minute core exercises is the limited intensity compared to longer, more traditional workouts. High-intensity exercise is essential for challenging the body, stimulating muscle growth, and improving cardiovascular fitness. However, with only five minutes to work with, it can be challenging to achieve the same level of intensity as a longer workout.

High-intensity exercise typically involves pushing the body to its limits, with short bursts of maximum effort followed by brief periods of rest or lower-intensity activity. This intensity is difficult to replicate in a short, 5-minute workout, where time constraints may limit the number of exercises performed or the duration of each exercise. As a result, individuals may struggle to achieve the same cardiovascular benefits and calorie burn as they would in a longer, more intense workout.

Additionally, limited intensity can impact the effectiveness of 5-minute core exercises for building strength and muscle mass. While short, high-intensity bursts can stimulate muscle growth and improve muscular endurance, the limited duration of 5-minute workouts may not provide enough stimulus to promote significant strength gains, especially for more advanced individuals.

To overcome the challenge of limited intensity in 5-minute core exercises, individuals can focus on maximizing effort and efficiency during each workout. By selecting compound exercises that engage multiple muscle groups simultaneously and incorporating interval training principles, individuals can increase the intensity of their workouts and maximize results in minimal time. Additionally, supplementing short core workouts with longer, more intense sessions periodically can help individuals achieve a balanced and comprehensive exercise routine.

Potential for Plateaus: Addressing the Need for Progressive Overload

Another disadvantage of 5-minute core exercises is the potential for plateaus in progress. Plateaus occur when the body adapts to a specific exercise routine and no longer experiences improvements in strength, endurance, or fitness. While plateaus are a natural part of the fitness journey, they can be particularly challenging to overcome with short, 5-minute workouts that may lack variety and progression.

Progressive overload is the key to continued progress and improvement in fitness. This principle involves gradually increasing the intensity, duration, or complexity of workouts over time to challenge the body and stimulate adaptation. However, with limited time and exercise options in a 5-minute workout, individuals may struggle to implement progressive overload effectively, leading to stagnation in progress and performance. Additionally, the repetitive nature of short, 5-minute workouts may contribute to plateaus by failing to provide adequate stimulus for continued growth and improvement. Without variation in exercises, intensity, or volume, the body may adapt quickly to the demands of the workout, resulting in diminished returns over time.

To address the potential for plateaus in 5-minute core exercises, individuals can incorporate strategies to promote progressive overload and variety in their workouts. This may include gradually increasing the intensity or duration of exercises, incorporating new exercises or equipment, adjusting rest periods, or changing the order or sequence of exercises to keep the body guessing and prevent adaptation.

Tailoring to Individual Needs: Adapting Exercises for Varied Fitness Levels

One of the challenges of 5-minute core exercises is the need to tailor workouts to individual fitness levels. While short workouts may be convenient and accessible for beginners or individuals with limited time, they may not provide enough challenge for more advanced individuals or those with specific fitness goals.

The effectiveness of 5-minute core exercises can vary widely depending on individual fitness levels, experience, and goals. For beginners, short workouts may provide a valuable introduction to core training and help establish a foundation of strength and stability. However, for more advanced individuals or those seeking specific fitness outcomes, such as muscle growth or sports performance enhancement, 5-minute workouts may not provide enough stimulus to achieve desired results.

Additionally, individuals with specific health concerns or limitations may require modifications or adaptations to 5-minute core exercises to ensure safety and effectiveness. For example, individuals with lower back pain or mobility issues may need to avoid certain exercises or perform modifications to reduce strain and discomfort.

To address the challenge of tailoring 5-minute core exercises to individual needs, individuals can focus on selecting exercises and modifications that align with their fitness level, goals, and limitations. This may involve consulting with a certified fitness professional or physical therapist to develop a personalized workout plan that addresses specific needs and concerns. Additionally, individuals can experiment with different exercises, variations, and modifications to find what works best for their body and goals. while 5-minute core exercises offer numerous benefits, including time-efficiency and accessibility, they also present certain disadvantages, such as limited intensity, potential for plateaus, and the need to tailor workouts to individual needs. By understanding these limitations and implementing strategies to overcome them, individuals can maximize the effectiveness of 5-minute core exercises and achieve their fitness goals in minimal time.

TIPS FOR MAXIMIZING RESULTS

Achieving optimal results from your core workouts requires more than just showing up and going through the motions. To truly maximize your efforts and see significant improvements in core strength, stability, and overall fitness, it's essential to approach your workouts with intention, strategy, and consistency. In this chapter, we'll explore key tips for maximizing results from your core exercises, including proper form and technique, supplementing with full-length workouts, and incorporating core exercises into your daily activities.

Proper Form and Technique: Ensuring Safe and Effective Workouts

One of the most critical aspects of any exercise routine is proper form and technique. Performing exercises with correct form not only maximizes the effectiveness of the workout but also reduces the risk of injury and ensures safe and sustainable progress over time. When it comes to core exercises, maintaining proper form is particularly important, as the core muscles play a central role in stabilizing the spine and supporting overall movement.

To ensure safe and effective core workouts, it's essential to focus on proper alignment, engagement, and execution of each exercise. Start by establishing a strong foundation with proper posture, ensuring that your spine is neutral, shoulders are relaxed, and core muscles are engaged. Throughout each exercise, pay attention to alignment cues, such as keeping the spine straight, hips level, and shoulders stacked over the wrists or elbows.

Additionally, focus on engaging the correct muscles and avoiding compensatory movements or reliance on other muscle groups. For example, during a plank exercise, focus on bracing the core muscles and avoiding excessive arching or rounding of the spine. Similarly, during a crunch or sit-up, focus on engaging the abdominal muscles and avoiding pulling on the neck or using momentum to lift the body.

Another essential aspect of proper form and technique is maintaining control throughout each movement and avoiding jerky or rapid motions. Slow, controlled movements not only increase the effectiveness of the exercise but also reduce the risk of injury by minimizing stress on the joints and connective tissues. Focus on smooth, controlled contractions of the core muscles, and avoid using momentum or gravity to power through the movement.

Finally, listen to your body and respect its limits. If you experience pain or discomfort during an exercise, stop immediately and reassess your form. It's better to perform exercises with proper form at a lower intensity than to risk injury by pushing through pain. Additionally, consider seeking guidance from a certified fitness professional or physical therapist to ensure that you're performing exercises correctly and safely.

Supplementing with Full-Length Workouts: Balancing Short Sessions with Longer Sessions

While 5-minute core exercises offer numerous benefits, they may not provide sufficient stimulus for certain fitness goals or individuals with specific needs. To maximize results and ensure a well-rounded exercise routine, it's essential to supplement short core sessions with longer, full-length workouts that target other muscle groups and fitness components.

Full-length workouts, typically ranging from 30 minutes to an hour or more, allow for more comprehensive training of the entire body, including the core, upper body, lower body, and cardiovascular system. These workouts provide an opportunity to incorporate a wider variety of exercises, equipment, and training modalities, resulting in greater muscle stimulation, calorie burn, and overall fitness improvements.

When supplementing short core sessions with full-length workouts, it's essential to prioritize balance and variety in your exercise routine. Incorporate a mix of strength training, cardiovascular exercise, and flexibility work to target different muscle groups and fitness components. For example, a full-length workout might include strength exercises such as squats, lunges, and push-ups, cardiovascular exercises such as running or cycling, and flexibility exercises such as yoga or stretching.

Additionally, consider the specific goals and needs of your fitness routine when designing full-length workouts. If your primary goal is to build strength and muscle mass, focus on incorporating compound exercises that target multiple muscle groups simultaneously, such as deadlifts, bench presses, and rows. If your goal is to improve cardiovascular fitness, prioritize exercises that elevate heart rate and challenge the cardiovascular system, such as running, cycling, or HIIT workouts.

It's also important to listen to your body and adjust the intensity and duration of full-length workouts based on your individual fitness level and recovery needs. While longer workouts can be beneficial for building endurance and promoting calorie burn, overtraining or pushing too hard can lead to fatigue, burnout, and increased risk of injury. Be mindful of signs of overtraining, such as persistent fatigue, soreness, or decreased performance, and give yourself permission to take rest days as needed.

Incorporating Core Exercises into Daily Activities

One of the most effective ways to maximize results from your core exercises is to incorporate them into your daily activities. While structured workouts are essential for building strength and fitness, the benefits of core training extend beyond the gym. By integrating core exercises into everyday movements and activities, you can strengthen your core muscles, improve posture and stability, and enhance overall functional fitness.

There are countless opportunities throughout the day to engage your core muscles and promote strength and stability. Whether you're sitting at your desk, standing in line at the grocery store, or walking the dog, there are simple exercises you can perform to activate your core and improve muscle engagement. For example, try drawing your navel toward your spine and engaging your abdominal muscles while sitting or standing, or practice maintaining a neutral spine and engaged core while walking or carrying objects.

In addition to integrating core exercises into everyday movements, consider incorporating dedicated core-focused activities into your daily routine. This might include setting aside a few minutes each morning or evening for a quick core workout, performing core exercises during commercial breaks while watching TV, or incorporating core-focused movements into household chores or gardening activities.

By making core training a consistent part of your daily routine, you can gradually build strength, stability, and endurance over time, leading to significant improvements in core health and overall fitness. Additionally, integrating core exercises into daily activities allows you to spread out your workout volume throughout the day, reducing the need for long, dedicated exercise sessions and making it easier to stay consistent with your fitness routine. maximizing results from your core exercises requires attention to proper form and technique, supplementation with full-length workouts, and integration into daily activities. By focusing on quality over quantity, balancing short core sessions with longer workouts, and incorporating core exercises into everyday movements, you can maximize the effectiveness of your workouts and achieve significant improvements in core strength, stability, and overall fitness. Remember to listen to your body, prioritize consistency, and celebrate progress along the way as you work towards your fitness goals.

ASSESSING YOUR CURRENT FITNESS LEVEL

Before diving headfirst into any new exercise routine, it's crucial to take stock of where you're starting from. Think of it as checking the map before embarking on a journey – you need to know where you are before you can plan where you're going. When it comes to assessing your current fitness level, there are a few key areas to consider.

First and foremost, take a moment to reflect on your overall health and any pre-existing medical conditions or injuries. Are there any physical limitations or restrictions that might affect your ability to exercise safely? If so, it's essential to consult with your healthcare provider before starting any new fitness regimen. They can provide valuable guidance tailored to your individual needs and help you navigate any potential obstacles along the way.

Next, consider your current level of physical activity. Are you a seasoned gym-goer with years of experience under your belt, or are you just dipping your toes into the world of fitness for the first time? Assessing your baseline level of activity can help you gauge where to start and set realistic goals for yourself.

Another important factor to consider is your flexibility, strength, and balance. These three components are key pillars of overall fitness and play a crucial role in core strength and stability. Take some time to evaluate your flexibility by performing simple stretches for major muscle groups like the hamstrings, quadriceps, and shoulders. Assess your strength by performing basic exercises like squats, lunges, and push-ups, taking note of how many repetitions you can comfortably complete. Finally, test your balance by standing on one leg with your eyes closed or performing a tandem stance (standing heel-to-toe) for a few seconds. Once you've completed your assessment, you'll have a clearer picture of where you stand and can tailor your exercise program accordingly. Remember, everyone's starting point is different, so don't compare yourself to others or feel discouraged if you're not where you want to be just yet. The important thing is to focus on progress, not perfection, and celebrate each small victory along the way.

Safety Precautions and Guidelines

When it comes to exercise, safety should always be your top priority. After all, there's nothing more counterproductive than getting injured and being sidelined from your workouts. That's why it's crucial to take some simple safety precautions before lacing up your sneakers and hitting the gym (or living room, if you prefer).

First and foremost, listen to your body. This might sound like common sense, but you'd be surprised how easy it is to ignore those subtle warning signs that something isn't quite right. If you experience any pain or discomfort during exercise, stop immediately and assess the situation. Pushing through the pain is never a good idea and can lead to further injury down the road.

Another important safety precaution is to start slowly and gradually increase the intensity of your workouts over time. Rome wasn't built in a day, and neither is a strong, healthy body. Trying to do too much, too soon is a recipe for disaster and can increase your risk of injury. Instead, start with lighter weights and fewer repetitions, focusing on perfecting your form and technique before adding more weight or increasing the intensity.

Proper form is another critical aspect of exercise safety, especially when it comes to core exercises. Performing exercises with improper form not only reduces their effectiveness but also increases your risk of injury. Take the time to learn the proper technique for each exercise and focus on maintaining good form throughout your workout. If you're unsure about how to perform a particular exercise, don't hesitate to ask a certified personal trainer or fitness instructor for guidance.

Finally, don't forget to stay hydrated and fuel your body with the nutrients it needs to perform at its best. Dehydration can impair your performance and increase your risk of injury, so be sure to drink plenty of water before, during, and after your workouts. And don't skimp on the fuel – your body needs a balanced diet rich in protein, carbohydrates, and healthy fats to support your active lifestyle.

Warm-up and Cool-down Exercises

You wouldn't start your car in the dead of winter without letting it warm up first, would you? The same principle applies to your body when it comes to exercise. Warming up before your workout helps prepare your muscles, joints, and cardiovascular system for the activity ahead, reducing your risk of injury and improving your performance.

A proper warm-up should include dynamic movements that increase blood flow to your muscles and joints, such as jogging in place, arm circles, leg swings, and hip rotations. Aim to spend at least 5-10 minutes warming up before diving into your main workout, gradually increasing the intensity as you go.

After your workout, don't forget to cool down and give your body a chance to recover. Cooling down helps lower your heart rate and prevent blood from pooling in your extremities, reducing the risk of dizziness or fainting. It also gives your muscles a chance to relax and can help prevent post-exercise soreness.

A typical cool-down routine might include gentle stretching exercises targeting the major muscle groups used during your workout, such as the quadriceps, hamstrings, calves, and shoulders. Hold each stretch for 15-30 seconds, breathing deeply and focusing on relaxing the muscles. And don't forget to hydrate – replenishing lost fluids is essential for recovery and helps flush out metabolic waste products from your muscles.

Getting started safely is the first step on your journey towards a stronger, healthier you. By assessing your current fitness level, taking simple safety precautions, and incorporating warm-up and cool-down exercises into your routine, you can minimize your risk of injury and set yourself up for long-term success. Remember, progress takes time, so be patient with yourself and enjoy the journey!

5-MINUTE CORE WORKOUTS

CORE EXERCISE BASICS

Welcome to the heart and soul of this book the 5-minute core workouts! If you're ready to strengthen your core, improve your stability, and boost your overall fitness in just a few short minutes a day, you're in the right place. But before we dive into the nitty-gritty of core exercises, let's start with the basics.

First and foremost, let's talk about what exactly constitutes a "core" exercise. While you might immediately think of crunches and planks, core exercises go far beyond these traditional moves. In fact, any exercise that engages the muscles of your abdomen, pelvis, lower back, and hips can be considered a core exercise. We're talking about movements like bridges, bird dogs, Russian twists, and so much more.

But here's the thing: when it comes to core exercises, quality always trumps quantity. It's not about how many reps you can crank out or how long you can hold a plank – it's about performing each exercise with proper form and technique to effectively engage your core muscles. Focus on maintaining a neutral spine, engaging your core muscles throughout the movement, and breathing deeply and rhythmically.

Another important aspect of core exercise is variety. Just like any other muscle group, your core muscles respond best to a diverse range of movements and stimuli. So don't be afraid to mix things up and try new exercises to challenge your core from all angles. From stability ball exercises to resistance band workouts, the possibilities are endless when it comes to core training.

Finally, consistency is key when it comes to seeing results from your core workouts. While it may be tempting to do a marathon session of crunches once a week and call it good, you'll see much better results by incorporating short, frequent workouts into your routine. That's where the beauty of the 5-minute core workout comes into play it's quick, convenient, and easy to squeeze into even the busiest of schedules.

So, whether you're a seasoned fitness enthusiast or a newcomer to the world of exercise, remember these core exercise basics as you embark on your journey towards a stronger, more resilient core. Focus on form, mix up your routine, and stay consistent you've got this!

Equipment Needed (Optional)

One of the best things about core exercises is that you don't need a lot of fancy equipment to get started. In fact, many effective core exercises can be done using nothing more than your own body weight. That being said, there are a few optional pieces of equipment that can add variety and intensity to your workouts if you so choose.

First up, we have the stability ball. Also known as an exercise ball or Swiss ball, this versatile piece of equipment can take your core workouts to the next level by adding an element of instability to your movements. Whether you're performing crunches, bridges, or planks, the stability ball forces your core muscles to work harder to maintain balance and stability, resulting in a more effective workout.

Next, we have resistance bands. These handy little bands come in a variety of shapes, sizes, and resistance levels, making them perfect for targeting your core muscles from all angles. Whether you're doing side bends, wood chops, or seated rows, resistance bands provide constant tension throughout the movement, helping to strengthen and tone your core muscles with every rep.

Other optional equipment for core workouts include medicine balls, kettlebells, and foam rollers, each offering unique benefits and challenges for your core muscles. However, it's important to remember that you can still get an effective core workout without any equipment at all – it's all about using what you have and getting creative with your exercises.

Sample 5-Minute Core Workout Routine

Now that you're familiar with the basics of core exercises and optional equipment, let's put it all together with a sample 5-minute core workout routine. This routine is designed to target all the major muscle groups of your core, including your abdominals, oblique's, and lower back, in just five short minutes.

- **Exercise 1:** Plank - 60 seconds Begin in a plank position with your hands directly under your shoulders and your body in a straight line from head to heels. Engage your core muscles and hold this position for 60 seconds, focusing on maintaining proper form and breathing deeply throughout the movement.

- **Exercise 2:** Russian Twists - 30 seconds Sit on the floor with your knees bent and your feet flat on the ground. Lean back slightly and lift your feet off the ground, balancing on your sit bones. Clasp your hands together in front of your chest and twist your torso to the right, then to the left, keeping your core engaged and your back straight. Continue alternating sides for 30 seconds.

- **Exercise 3:** Bicycle Crunches - 45 seconds Lie on your back with your knees bent and your hands behind your head. Lift your head, neck, and shoulders off the ground and bring your right elbow towards your left knee while straightening your right leg. Switch sides, bringing your left elbow towards your right knee while straightening your left leg. Continue alternating sides in a fluid, bicycle-like motion for 45 seconds.

- **Exercise 4:** Bird Dogs - 60 seconds Begin on your hands and knees with your wrists directly under your shoulders and your knees directly under your hips. Extend your right arm forward and your left leg back, keeping your core engaged and your back flat. Hold this position for a few seconds, then return to the starting position and switch sides. Continue alternating sides for 60 seconds, focusing on stability and control.

- **Exercise 5:** Bridge - 45 seconds Lie on your back with your knees bent and your feet flat on the ground. Press through your heels to lift your hips off the ground, forming a straight line from your shoulders to your knees. Squeeze your glutes and engage your core as you hold this position for 45 seconds, then lower your hips back down to the ground.

Congratulations you've completed your 5-minute core workout! Repeat this routine 2-3 times for a complete core workout that will leave you feeling strong, stable, and energized. And remember, consistency is key when it comes to seeing results, so try to incorporate this workout into your routine 3-5 times per week for best results.

With these core exercise basics, optional equipment suggestions, and a sample 5-minute workout routine in your arsenal, you're well-equipped to start strengthening your core and reaping the countless benefits that come with it. So grab your mat, lace up your sneakers, and let's get to work your core will thank you!

CORE EXERCISES FOR SENIORS

As we age, maintaining a strong and stable core becomes increasingly important for overall health and well-being. A strong core not only helps improve posture and balance but also reduces the risk of falls and supports daily activities. In this chapter, we'll explore a variety of core exercises specifically tailored for seniors, focusing on seated, standing, resistance band, and balance and stability exercises.

Seated Core Exercises

For seniors who may have mobility limitations or prefer exercising from a seated position, seated core exercises offer a safe and effective way to strengthen the core muscles. These exercises can be performed in a chair or wheelchair and target key muscle groups without putting undue stress on the joints. Here are some seated core exercises to try:

- **Seated Marching:** Sit tall in a chair with your feet flat on the ground. Lift one knee towards your chest, then lower it back down and repeat with the other leg. Alternate between legs in a marching motion, engaging your core muscles to maintain stability.

- **Seated Side Bends:** Sit tall in a chair with your feet flat on the ground and your hands resting on your thighs. Inhale to lengthen your spine, then exhale as you gently lean to one side, reaching towards the floor with your hand. Return to the starting position and repeat on the other side, focusing on stretching and strengthening the oblique muscles.

- **Seated Torso Twists:** Sit tall in a chair with your feet flat on the ground and your hands clasped together in front of your chest. Inhale to lengthen your spine, then exhale as you twist your torso to one side, keeping your hips square. Return to the center and repeat on the other side, engaging your core muscles throughout the movement.

- **Seated Leg Raises:** Sit tall in a chair with your feet flat on the ground and your hands resting on the sides of the chair for support. Lift one leg off the ground, extending it straight out in front of you, then lower it back down and repeat with the other leg. Engage your core muscles to stabilize your body throughout the movement.

Standing Core Exercises

For seniors who are able to stand comfortably, standing core exercises offer a great way to improve balance, stability, and overall strength. These exercises engage multiple muscle groups simultaneously, helping to strengthen the core while also improving coordination and mobility. Here are some standing core exercises to try:

- **Standing Marches:** Stand tall with your feet hip-width apart and your arms by your sides. Lift one knee towards your chest, then lower it back down and repeat with the other leg. Alternate between legs in a marching motion, engaging your core muscles to maintain balance and stability.

- **Standing Side Bends:** Stand tall with your feet hip-width apart and your arms extended overhead. Inhale to lengthen your spine, then exhale as you gently lean to one side, reaching towards the floor with your hand. Return to the center and repeat on the other side, focusing on stretching and strengthening the oblique muscles.

- **Standing Torso Twists:** Stand tall with your feet hip-width apart and your arms extended straight out in front of you. Inhale to prepare, then exhale as you twist your torso to one side, keeping your hips square. Return to the center and repeat on the other side, engaging your core muscles throughout the movement.

- **Standing Leg Raises:** Stand tall with your feet hip-width apart and your hands resting on a stable surface for support. Lift one leg out to the side, keeping it straight and engaged, then lower it back down and repeat with the other leg. Focus on engaging your core muscles to maintain stability throughout the movement.

Core Exercises with Resistance Bands

Resistance bands are a versatile and effective tool for adding resistance to core exercises, making them more challenging and engaging. For seniors looking to increase strength and stability in their core muscles, resistance band exercises offer a safe and convenient option. Here are some core exercises with resistance bands to try:

- **Seated Row:** Sit tall in a chair with your feet flat on the ground and a resistance band looped around your feet. Hold onto the ends of the resistance band with both hands, palms facing each other. Engage your core muscles and exhale as you pull the resistance band towards your chest, squeezing your shoulder blades together. Inhale to return to the starting position and repeat for several repetitions.

- **Standing Wood Chop:** Stand tall with your feet hip-width apart and a resistance band anchored at shoulder height to your side. Hold onto the end of the resistance band with both hands, arms extended straight out in front of you. Engage your core muscles and exhale as you rotate your torso and pull the resistance band diagonally across your body, ending with your hands above your opposite shoulder. Inhale to return to the starting position and repeat on the other side.

- **Side Leg Lifts:** Attach a resistance band around your ankles and stand tall with your feet hip-width apart. Engage your core muscles and exhale as you lift one leg out to the side against the resistance of the band, keeping it straight and engaged. Inhale to return to the starting position and repeat on the other side.

- **Pallof Press:** Attach a resistance band to a sturdy anchor point at chest height and stand sideways to the anchor point with the band in both hands. Engage your core muscles and exhale as you press the resistance band straight out in front of you, extending your arms fully. Hold for a moment, then inhale to return to the starting position and repeat for several repetitions.

Balance and Stability Exercises

Maintaining good balance and stability is essential for preventing falls and maintaining independence as we age. Fortunately, there are a variety of balance and stability exercises that target the core muscles and improve overall stability. Here are some balance and stability exercises for seniors:

- **Single Leg Balance:** Stand tall with your feet hip-width apart and your hands on your hips. Shift your weight onto one leg and lift the other leg off the ground, balancing on the standing leg. Engage your core muscles and hold this position for 30 seconds to 1 minute, then switch sides.

- **Heel-to-Toe Walk:** Stand tall with your feet together and your arms by your sides. Take a step forward with one foot, placing it directly in front of the other foot so that the heel of the front foot touches the toes of the back foot. Continue walking in a straight line, placing one foot directly in front of the other, for 10-20 steps.

- **Balance Board Exercises:** Stand on a balance board or wobble board with your feet hip-width apart and your core engaged. Practice maintaining your balance on the board by shifting your weight from side to side and front to back. As you become more comfortable, try performing exercises such as squats or single-leg balances on the board.

- **Tai Chi:** Tai Chi is a gentle form of exercise that focuses on slow, flowing movements and deep breathing. It has been shown to improve balance, flexibility, and strength, making it an excellent choice for seniors looking to improve their core stability. Consider taking a Tai Chi class or following along with instructional videos online.

These core exercises for seniors are designed to improve strength, stability, and overall health in a safe and effective manner. Whether you're exercising from a seated or standing position, using resistance bands, or focusing on balance and stability, incorporating these exercises into your routine can help you maintain independence and vitality well into your golden years. Remember to start slowly, listen to your body, and consult with a healthcare professional before beginning any new exercise program.

PROGRESSING YOUR CORE WORKOUTS

As you continue on your journey to strengthen your core and improve your overall fitness, it's important to keep challenging yourself and progressing your workouts over time. In this chapter, we'll explore strategies for increasing the intensity of your core workouts safely, tracking your progress, and modifying exercises to meet your individual needs.

Increasing Intensity Safely

As you become more experienced with core exercises, you may find that your workouts start to feel easier or less challenging. This is a sign that it's time to increase the intensity of your workouts to continue seeing progress. However, it's important to do so safely and gradually to avoid injury. Here are some tips for increasing the intensity of your core workouts safely:

- **Increase Repetitions or Sets:** One simple way to increase the intensity of your core workouts is to perform more repetitions or sets of each exercise. For example, if you've been doing 10 repetitions of each exercise, try increasing to 15 or 20 repetitions, or adding an additional set.

- **Decrease Rest Time:** Another way to ramp up the intensity of your workouts is to decrease the rest time between exercises or sets. Instead of taking a full minute of rest between sets, try reducing it to 30 seconds or even eliminating rest periods altogether for a more challenging workout.

- **Add Resistance:** Adding resistance to your core exercises is a great way to increase the intensity and stimulate further muscle growth. You can do this by using resistance bands, dumbbells, or other weighted equipment to make the exercises more challenging. For example, you can hold a dumbbell or medicine ball while performing exercises like Russian twists or wood chops.

- **Progress to Advanced Variations:** As you become more proficient with basic core exercises, consider progressing to more advanced variations to further challenge your muscles. For example, you can advance from regular planks to side planks, or from bicycle crunches to hanging leg raises. Just be sure to maintain proper form and technique to avoid injury.

- **Incorporate Plyometric:** Plyometric exercises, which involve explosive movements like jumps and hops, are another excellent way to increase the intensity of your core workouts. Plyometric exercises engage multiple muscle groups simultaneously and can help improve power, strength, and agility.

Remember, the key to increasing the intensity of your core workouts safely is to do so gradually and listen to your body. Pay attention to how your muscles feel during and after your workouts, and don't push yourself beyond your limits. If you experience any pain or discomfort, scale back the intensity or take a break to allow your body to recover.

Tracking Your Progress

Tracking your progress is essential for staying motivated and ensuring that you're making consistent gains in your core strength and fitness. By keeping track of key metrics such as repetitions, sets, weight lifted, and workout duration, you can monitor your progress over time and make adjustments as needed. Here are some tips for effectively tracking your progress:

- **Keep a Workout Journal:** One of the simplest and most effective ways to track your progress is to keep a workout journal or log. Write down details of each workout, including the exercises performed, number of repetitions and sets, weight lifted, and any notes or observations. This will allow you to see how your strength and endurance improve over time.

- **Use Fitness Apps or Trackers:** There are countless fitness apps and trackers available that can help you monitor your workouts and progress. These apps allow you to input details of each workout, track your performance over time, and set goals for yourself. Some apps even offer personalized workout plans and progress reports to help keep you on track.

- **Take Progress Photos:** Another useful tool for tracking your progress is to take regular progress photos. Take photos of yourself from different angles at the beginning of your fitness journey, then take new photos every few weeks or months to compare. This visual representation of your progress can be incredibly motivating and rewarding.

- **Measure Functional Fitness:** In addition to tracking traditional metrics like repetitions and sets, consider measuring functional fitness markers such as balance, flexibility, and mobility. Keep track of how long you can hold a plank, how far you can reach in a seated forward fold, or how easily you can perform daily activities like getting up from a chair or climbing stairs.

- **Celebrate Milestones:** Finally, don't forget to celebrate your progress and milestones along the way. Whether it's reaching a new personal best in a particular exercise, completing a full set of advanced variations, or simply feeling stronger and more energized in your daily life, take the time to acknowledge and celebrate your achievements.

Modifying Exercises for Individual Needs

One of the great things about core exercises is that they can be easily modified to meet individual needs and abilities. Whether you're recovering from an injury, dealing with a chronic condition, or simply looking for ways to tailor your workouts to your unique body, there are plenty of options available. Here are some tips for modifying core exercises to meet your individual needs:

- **Focus on Form and Technique:** Regardless of your fitness level or ability, proper form and technique should always be a top priority. Focus on performing each exercise with controlled, deliberate movements and engaging the correct muscles throughout. If you're unsure about how to perform a particular exercise, don't hesitate to ask a certified personal trainer or fitness instructor for guidance.

- **Use Props or Modifications:** If you have mobility limitations or physical restrictions, don't be afraid to use props or modifications to make exercises more accessible. For example, you can use a chair or wall for support during standing exercises, or modify exercises like planks or bridges by performing them from a kneeling or seated position.

- **Listen to Your Body:** Above all, listen to your body and honor its needs and limitations. If you experience any pain or discomfort during exercise, stop immediately and assess the situation. It's better to scale back the intensity or modify the exercise than to risk injury by pushing through pain.

- **Work with a Professional:** If you have specific health concerns or medical conditions, consider working with a certified personal trainer or physical therapist who can create a customized workout plan tailored to your individual needs. They can help you identify any potential limitations or areas for improvement and provide guidance and support every step of the way.

Remember, the most important thing is to find exercises that feel safe and comfortable for your body, and to listen to your body's signals during your workouts. With a little creativity and flexibility, you can modify core exercises to meet your individual needs and continue making progress towards your fitness goals.

By safely increasing the intensity of your core workouts, tracking your progress, and modifying exercises to meet your individual needs, you can continue to challenge yourself and see consistent gains in core strength and overall fitness. Whether you're a beginner or a seasoned fitness enthusiast, these strategies will help you stay on track and achieve your goals.

INCORPORATING CORE EXERCISES INTO DAILY LIFE

Incorporating core exercises into your daily life is one of the most effective ways to strengthen your core muscles and improve overall health and fitness. By integrating core workouts into your routine, you can reap the benefits of increased stability, better posture, and reduced risk of injury, all without needing to set aside dedicated time for a separate workout session. In this chapter, we'll explore strategies for seamlessly integrating core exercises into your daily life, staying consistent with your routine, and overcoming common barriers that may arise along the way.

Integrating Core Workouts into Your Routine

The key to incorporating core exercises into your daily life is to find simple and convenient ways to sneak them into your existing routine. By making small adjustments and being intentional about how you move throughout the day, you can effectively target your core muscles without needing to carve out extra time for formal exercise. Here are some tips for integrating core workouts into your routine:

- **Practice Good Posture:** Believe it or not, something as simple as sitting or standing with good posture can engage your core muscles and provide a subtle workout throughout the day. Focus on sitting up tall, keeping your shoulders back and down, and engaging your abdominal muscles to support your spine. Whether you're at your desk, in the car, or standing in line at the grocery store, take advantage of every opportunity to practice good posture and engage your core.

- **Incorporate Core Exercises into Daily Activities:** Look for opportunities to incorporate core exercises into activities you're already doing throughout the day. For example, try doing a few standing leg raises while brushing your teeth, or perform seated torso twists while waiting for the kettle to boil. By multitasking and combining core exercises with daily activities, you can sneak in extra repetitions without needing to set aside dedicated workout time.

- **Take Active Breaks:** Instead of sitting for long periods, take regular breaks to move and stretch your body. Set a timer to remind yourself to get up and move around every hour, and use this time to perform a quick set of core exercises such as planks, squats, or lunges. Not only will this help keep your muscles engaged and your energy levels up, but it can also improve circulation and reduce stiffness and discomfort from prolonged sitting.

- **Make Household Chores Count:** Household chores offer countless opportunities to engage your core muscles and get in a workout while completing everyday tasks. Whether you're vacuuming, mopping, gardening, or doing laundry, focus on using your core muscles to support your movements and maintain proper form. For example, engage your core and squat down to lift heavy objects instead of bending at the waist, or tighten your abdominal muscles while carrying groceries up the stairs.

- **Embrace Active Transportation:** Whenever possible, opt for active modes of transportation that require physical effort and engage your core muscles. Consider walking or biking to work instead of driving, taking the stairs instead of the elevator, or parking farther away from your destination to incorporate more movement into your day. Not only will you save money on gas and reduce your carbon footprint, but you'll also sneak in a mini-workout along the way.

By finding creative ways to integrate core exercises into your daily life, you can effectively target your core muscles and improve overall strength and stability without needing to set aside dedicated workout time. Whether you're sitting at your desk, running errands, or doing household chores, there are countless opportunities to engage your core and reap the benefits of regular exercise.

Tips for Staying Consistent

Consistency is key when it comes to incorporating core exercises into your daily life. While it's easy to get excited and motivated to start a new routine, staying consistent over the long term can be challenging. Fortunately, there are several strategies you can use to help stay on track and make core exercises a regular part of your daily routine. Here are some tips for staying consistent:

- **Set Realistic Goals:** Start by setting realistic, achievable goals for yourself when it comes to incorporating core exercises into your daily life. Instead of aiming to do a full hour of core exercises every day, start small with just a few minutes of core work each day and gradually increase the duration and intensity over time. Setting realistic goals will help you stay motivated and avoid burnout.

- **Schedule it in:** Treat core exercises like any other important appointment or commitment by scheduling them into your daily routine. Whether it's first thing in the morning, during your lunch break, or before bed, set aside dedicated time each day to focus on core exercises. By making it a non-negotiable part of your schedule, you're more likely to stick with it over the long term.

- **Find an Accountability Partner:** Enlist the support of a friend, family member, or workout buddy to help hold you accountable and stay motivated. Share your goals with them and check in regularly to update them on your progress. Knowing that someone else is counting on you can provide an extra incentive to stay consistent and stick to your routine.

- **Mix it Up:** Keep your core workouts interesting and engaging by mixing up your routine and trying new exercises regularly. Incorporate a variety of core exercises targeting different muscle groups, and experiment with different formats such as circuit training, interval training, or bodyweight exercises. Not only will this help prevent boredom, but it will also keep your muscles guessing and promote continued progress.

- **Celebrate Your Successes:** Don't forget to celebrate your successes and milestones along the way. Whether it's reaching a new personal best in a particular exercise, sticking to your routine for a full week, or simply feeling stronger and more energized, take the time to acknowledge and celebrate your achievements.

Positive reinforcement can help reinforce your commitment and motivate you to keep going.

By setting realistic goals, scheduling core exercises into your daily routine, finding an accountability partner, mixing up your workouts, and celebrating your successes, you can stay consistent and make core exercises a regular part of your daily life. Remember, consistency is key when it comes to seeing results, so stick with it and keep pushing forward.

Overcoming Common Barriers

Despite your best intentions, you may encounter obstacles and challenges along the way that threaten to derail your efforts to incorporate core exercises into your daily life. From busy schedules to lack of motivation, these barriers can make it difficult to stay consistent with your routine. However, with some planning and determination, you can overcome these common barriers and stay on track towards your fitness goals. Here are some strategies for overcoming common barriers:

- **Lack of Time:** One of the most common barriers to regular exercise is a perceived lack of time. However, with a little creativity and planning, you can find ways to squeeze in core exercises throughout your day. Look for small pockets of time in your schedule, such as during TV commercials, while waiting for dinner to cook, or during your lunch break, and use these opportunities to sneak in a quick workout.

- **Lack of Motivation:** Another common barrier to regular exercise is a lack of motivation, especially when you're tired or busy. To overcome this barrier, try finding activities that you enjoy and look forward to, whether it's going for a walk in nature, dancing to your favorite music, or practicing yoga. Remember that exercise doesn't have to be a chore – it can be fun and enjoyable, too.

- **Lack of Resources:** If you don't have access to a gym or exercise equipment, it can be challenging to stay consistent with your workouts. However, there are plenty of bodyweight exercises and household items that you can use to create an effective workout at home. Get creative with your surroundings and use everyday objects like chairs, water bottles, or towels to add resistance and challenge to your workouts.

- **Lack of Support:** Having a strong support system can make all the difference when it comes to sticking to your fitness goals. If you're feeling unsupported or discouraged, reach out to friends, family members, or online communities for encouragement and motivation. Surround yourself with people who believe in you and want to see you succeed, and don't be afraid to ask for help when you need it.

- **Fear of Injury:** Fear of injury can be a major barrier to starting or sticking with a regular exercise routine, especially for seniors or those with existing health concerns. To overcome this barrier, start slowly and gradually increase the intensity of your workouts as your strength and confidence grow. Focus on proper form and technique, listen to your body, and don't push yourself beyond your limits. If you're unsure about how to perform a particular exercise safely, seek guidance from a certified personal trainer or fitness professional.

By identifying common barriers and implementing strategies to overcome them, you can stay consistent with your core exercises and make regular physical activity a priority in your daily life. Remember that consistency is key when it comes to seeing results, so stay focused, stay positive, and keep pushing forward.

NUTRITION AND CORE HEALTH

Nutrition plays a critical role in overall health and well-being, and this holds true for core strength as well. In this chapter, we'll delve into the importance of nutrition for core strength, explore foods that support core health, and discuss hydration tips for optimal performance.

Importance of Nutrition for Core Strength

When it comes to building a strong and resilient core, nutrition is just as important as exercise. Your core muscles rely on a steady supply of nutrients to function properly, repair tissue damage, and recover from workouts. A well-balanced diet provides the essential vitamins, minerals, and macronutrients necessary to support muscle growth, repair, and maintenance.

Protein is especially important for core health, as it provides the building blocks necessary for muscle repair and growth. Aim to include a source of lean protein with every meal, such as chicken, turkey, fish, tofu, beans, or lentils. Additionally, consuming an adequate amount of carbohydrates provides the energy needed to fuel your workouts and support optimal performance. Choose complex carbohydrates like whole grains, fruits, vegetables, and legumes to provide sustained energy throughout the day.

Healthy fats are another essential component of a balanced diet and play a crucial role in supporting overall health and vitality. Omega-3 fatty acids, found in fatty fish, flaxseeds, chia seeds, and walnuts, have anti-inflammatory properties that can help reduce muscle soreness and promote faster recovery. Incorporating a variety of colorful fruits and vegetables into your diet provides essential vitamins, minerals, and antioxidants that support overall health and immune function.

In addition to macronutrients, hydration is also essential for optimal core health. Dehydration can impair muscle function and performance, making it harder to engage your core muscles effectively during workouts. Aim to drink plenty of water throughout the day, especially before, during, and after exercise, to stay properly hydrated and support optimal performance.

Foods that Support Core Health

Incorporating nutrient-rich foods into your diet is essential for supporting core health and function. Here are some foods that can help support a strong and resilient core:

- **Greek Yogurt:** Greek yogurt is an excellent source of protein, calcium, and probiotics, making it a great choice for supporting overall muscle health and digestion. Enjoy it as a snack or add it to smoothies and parfaits for a creamy and nutritious boost.
- **Leafy Greens:** Leafy greens like spinach, kale, and Swiss chard are packed with vitamins, minerals, and antioxidants that support overall health and well-being. They're also low in calories and high in fiber, making them an excellent choice for promoting satiety and weight management.
- **Berries:** Berries like strawberries, blueberries, and raspberries are rich in antioxidants and anti-inflammatory compounds that can help reduce muscle soreness and inflammation. Enjoy them fresh or frozen as a topping for oatmeal, yogurt, or salads.

- **Salmon:** Salmon is an excellent source of protein and omega-3 fatty acids, which have been shown to reduce inflammation, improve muscle recovery, and support overall heart health. Aim to include fatty fish like salmon, mackerel, and sardines in your diet at least twice a week.

- **Nuts and Seeds:** Nuts and seeds like almonds, walnuts, chia seeds, and flaxseeds are rich in healthy fats, protein, and fiber, making them a nutritious and satisfying snack option. Sprinkle them on salads, yogurt, or oatmeal for an extra boost of nutrients and flavor.

- **Whole Grains:** Whole grains like quinoa, brown rice, oats, and barley are rich in complex carbohydrates, which provide sustained energy and support optimal performance during workouts. Swap refined grains like white bread and pasta for whole grains to promote satiety and support overall health.

- **Lean Protein:** Lean protein sources like chicken, turkey, fish, tofu, beans, and lentils are essential for supporting muscle repair and growth. Aim to include a source of lean protein with every meal to support optimal core health and function.

Hydration Tips for Optimal Performance

Proper hydration is essential for maintaining optimal core health and supporting peak performance during workouts. Dehydration can impair muscle function, reduce endurance, and increase the risk of cramps and injury. Here are some hydration tips to help you stay properly hydrated and perform at your best:

- **Drink Water Regularly:** Aim to drink water regularly throughout the day, especially before, during, and after exercise. Carry a reusable water bottle with you and take sips frequently to stay hydrated.

- **Monitor Urine Color:** Pay attention to the color of your urine as a simple indicator of hydration status. Ideally, your urine should be pale yellow in color. Dark yellow or amber-colored urine may indicate dehydration and a need to drink more fluids.

- **Consider Electrolyte Replacement:** If you're engaging in prolonged or intense exercise, consider replenishing electrolytes lost through sweat with sports drinks or electrolyte tablets. Electrolytes like sodium, potassium, and magnesium play a crucial role in maintaining fluid balance and muscle function.

- **Eat Water-Rich Foods:** In addition to drinking water, incorporate water-rich foods like fruits and vegetables into your diet to help meet your hydration needs. Foods like watermelon, cucumber, celery, and oranges have high water content and can help contribute to your overall fluid intake.

- **Listen to Your Body:** Pay attention to how your body feels during exercise and adjust your fluid intake accordingly. If you're feeling thirsty, fatigued, or experiencing muscle cramps, it may be a sign that you need to drink more fluids.

- **Plan Ahead:** Be proactive about staying hydrated by planning ahead and ensuring you have access to water or electrolyte beverages during workouts and throughout the day. Fill up your water bottle before leaving the house and make hydration a priority during exercise.

- **Avoid Excessive Caffeine and Alcohol:** Limit your intake of caffeine and alcohol, as both can have diuretic effects and contribute to dehydration. If you do consume caffeinated or alcoholic beverages, be sure to drink water as well to offset their dehydrating effects.

By incorporating nutrient-rich foods into your diet, staying properly hydrated, and paying attention to your body's hydration needs, you can support optimal core health and performance. Remember to focus on whole, minimally processed foods, stay hydrated throughout the day, and listen to your body's signals to ensure you're meeting your nutritional needs.

nutrition plays a crucial role in supporting core health and function. By consuming a well-balanced diet rich in lean protein, healthy fats, complex carbohydrates, fruits, vegetables, and plenty of water, you can provide your body with the essential nutrients it needs to build and maintain a strong and resilient core. Whether you're fueling up for a workout, recovering from exercise, or simply nourishing your body for overall health and well-being, prioritize nutrient-rich foods and hydration to support optimal core health and performance.

COMMON CHALLENGES AND SOLUTIONS

Embarking on a journey to improve core strength and overall fitness is a commendable endeavor, but it's not without its challenges. In this chapter, we'll explore common challenges faced by individuals striving to enhance their core health and provide practical solutions to overcome these obstacles.

Dealing with Soreness and Injury Prevention

One of the most common challenges encountered when starting or increasing core workouts is dealing with soreness. Soreness, also known as delayed onset muscle soreness (DOMS), typically occurs 24 to 48 hours after exercise and can range from mild discomfort to significant pain. While some degree of soreness is normal and indicates that your muscles are adapting to the demands of exercise, excessive soreness can interfere with your ability to perform daily activities and hinder your progress. Here are some strategies to deal with soreness and prevent injury:

- **Gradually Increase Intensity:** One of the most effective ways to prevent soreness and injury is to gradually increase the intensity and duration of your workouts over time. Start with lighter weights and fewer repetitions and gradually increase as your strength and endurance improve. This allows your muscles to adapt gradually to the increased demands placed on them, reducing the risk of soreness and injury.

- **Warm-Up and Cool Down Properly:** Proper warm-up and cool-down routines are essential for preparing your muscles for exercise and aiding in recovery afterward. Before starting your workout, spend 5-10 minutes performing dynamic stretches and light cardio exercises to increase blood flow and loosen up your muscles. Afterward, take another 5-10 minutes to perform static stretches and gentle mobility exercises to help your muscles relax and recover.

- **Focus on Form and Technique:** Proper form and technique are crucial for preventing injuries and minimizing soreness during exercise. Focus on maintaining good posture and alignment throughout your workouts, and pay attention to cues from your body. If you experience any sharp or sudden pain during exercise, stop immediately and reassess your form. It's better to perform exercises correctly with lighter weights than to risk injury by using improper form with heavier weights.

- **Listen to Your Body:** One of the most important things you can do to prevent soreness and injury is to listen to your body and respect its limits. If you're feeling overly fatigued or experiencing excessive soreness, it's okay to take a break or scale back the intensity of your workouts. Pushing through pain or fatigue can increase the risk of injury and delay recovery, so prioritize rest and recovery when needed.

- **Incorporate Recovery Strategies:** In addition to proper warm-up and cool-down routines, incorporating other recovery strategies can help minimize soreness and support muscle recovery. Consider incorporating activities like foam rolling, massage, stretching, and restorative yoga into your routine to help alleviate muscle tension and promote relaxation.

By implementing these strategies, you can effectively deal with soreness and prevent injury, allowing you to continue making progress towards your core strength and fitness goals.

Motivation Strategies for Consistent Workouts

Another common challenge faced by individuals striving to improve core health is maintaining motivation for consistent workouts. It's easy to get excited and motivated when starting a new fitness routine, but staying consistent over the long term can be challenging. Here are some strategies to help you stay motivated and committed to your workouts:

- **Set Realistic Goals:** Start by setting realistic, achievable goals for yourself that align with your core health and fitness objectives. Whether it's improving core strength, increasing endurance, or achieving a specific fitness milestone, having clear goals can provide direction and motivation for your workouts.

- **Find Your Why:** Take some time to reflect on why improving your core health is important to you and what motivates you to stay committed to your fitness routine. Whether it's improving overall health and well-being, reducing pain and discomfort, or increasing confidence and vitality, identifying your underlying motivations can help fuel your commitment and dedication.

- **Create a Supportive Environment:** Surround yourself with people who support and encourage your fitness goals, whether it's friends, family members, or workout buddies. Having a supportive network can provide accountability, motivation, and camaraderie, making it easier to stay consistent with your workouts.

- **Mix Up Your Routine:** Keep your workouts interesting and engaging by mixing up your routine and trying new activities or exercises regularly. Incorporate a variety of exercises targeting different muscle groups, and experiment with different formats such as circuit training, interval training, or group classes. Not only will this prevent boredom, but it will also keep your muscles guessing and promote continued progress.

- **Schedule it in:** Treat your workouts like any other important appointment or commitment by scheduling them into your daily or weekly routine. Set aside dedicated time for exercise and prioritize it just like you would any other task. By making exercise a non-negotiable part of your schedule, you're more likely to stick with it over the long term.

- **Celebrate Your Progress:** Take time to celebrate your progress and achievements along the way, no matter how small they may seem. Whether it's reaching a new personal best in a particular exercise, completing a full week of consistent workouts, or simply feeling stronger and more energized, acknowledge and celebrate your successes to stay motivated and inspired.

By implementing these motivation strategies, you can stay consistent with your workouts and maintain momentum towards your core health and fitness goals.

Overcoming Plateaus and Stagnation

Even with the best intentions and efforts, it's common to experience plateaus and stagnation in your fitness journey. Plateaus occur when your progress slows or stalls, despite consistent effort and dedication to your workouts. While frustrating, plateaus are a normal part of the fitness journey and can be overcome with the right approach. Here are some strategies to help you overcome plateaus and continue making progress towards your core health and fitness goals:

- **Mix Up Your Workouts:** If you've been following the same workout routine for an extended period, it's possible that your body has adapted to the stimulus, leading to a plateau in progress. Mix things up by incorporating new exercises, changing the order or intensity of your workouts, or trying a different fitness format altogether. This can challenge your muscles in new ways and stimulate further growth and adaptation.

- **Increase Intensity or Volume:** To continue making progress, consider increasing the intensity or volume of your workouts. This can be achieved by adding more weight, increasing the number of repetitions or sets, shortening rest periods between exercises, or incorporating more challenging variations of existing exercises. By progressively overloading your muscles, you can continue to challenge them and stimulate growth.

- **Focus on Recovery:** Adequate rest and recovery are essential for overcoming plateaus and promoting muscle growth and adaptation. Make sure you're prioritizing sleep, nutrition, hydration, and stress management to support optimal recovery between workouts. Incorporate rest days into your routine as needed, and listen to your body's signals to avoid overtraining and burnout.

- **Set New Goals:** Reassess your goals and set new targets to keep yourself motivated and focused. Whether it's increasing the duration of your plank hold, lifting heavier weights, or mastering a new exercise variation, having clear goals can provide direction and purpose for your workouts. Break larger goals down into smaller, achievable milestones, and celebrate your progress along the way.

- **Seek Professional Guidance:** If you're struggling to overcome a plateau or stagnation in your fitness journey, consider seeking guidance from a certified personal trainer or fitness professional. They can assess your current routine, identify areas for improvement, and create a customized workout plan tailored to your individual needs and goals. Working with a professional can provide accountability, support, and guidance to help you break through barriers and reach new heights in your fitness journey.

By implementing these strategies, you can overcome plateaus and stagnation in your fitness journey, continue making progress towards your core health and fitness goals, and achieve lasting results. common challenges such as dealing with soreness, maintaining motivation, and overcoming plateaus are all normal aspects of the fitness journey. By implementing practical solutions such as proper warm-up and cool-down routines, setting realistic goals, staying accountable, mixing up your workouts, and seeking professional guidance when needed, you can overcome these obstacles and continue making progress towards your core health and fitness goals. Remember to listen to your body, stay patient and persistent, and celebrate your successes along the way. With dedication, determination, and the right mindset, you can overcome any challenge and achieve the strong and resilient core you desire.

SPECIAL CONSIDERATIONS FOR SENIORS

As we age, maintaining core strength and overall fitness becomes increasingly important for preserving independence, mobility, and quality of life. However, seniors may face unique challenges and considerations when it comes to engaging in core exercises. In this chapter, we'll explore special considerations for seniors, including adapting core exercises for joint health, addressing mobility issues, and consulting with healthcare professionals for personalized guidance and support.

Adapting Core Exercises for Joint Health

Joint health is a critical consideration for seniors when engaging in core exercises. As we age, our joints may become stiffer, less flexible, and more prone to pain and discomfort. It's essential to choose core exercises that are gentle on the joints while still effective for strengthening the core muscles. Here are some tips for adapting core exercises for joint health:

- **Focus on Low-Impact Exercises:** Opt for low-impact core exercises that minimize stress on the joints while still providing a challenging workout. Examples of low-impact exercises include seated core exercises, gentle stretching, and movements performed in a controlled range of motion. Avoid high-impact exercises like jumping or running, which can exacerbate joint pain and discomfort.

- **Use Proper Form and Technique:** Proper form and technique are crucial for protecting the joints and preventing injury during core exercises. Focus on maintaining good posture and alignment throughout each exercise, and avoid any movements that cause pain or discomfort. If you're unsure about how to perform a particular exercise safely, consider working with a certified personal trainer or physical therapist for guidance.

- **Choose Joint-Friendly Equipment:** When incorporating equipment into your core workouts, choose options that are gentle on the joints. For example, consider using resistance bands, stability balls, or foam rollers instead of heavy weights or machines. These tools provide resistance without putting undue stress on the joints, making them suitable for seniors with joint issues.

- **Listen to Your Body:** Pay attention to how your body responds to different exercises and movements, and adjust accordingly. If you experience any pain, discomfort, or instability during exercise, stop immediately and reassess your approach. It's essential to listen to your body's signals and respect its limits to prevent further injury and promote joint health.

- **Incorporate Range-of-Motion Exercises:** Include exercises that focus on improving joint flexibility and range of motion in your core workout routine. Gentle movements like shoulder rolls, hip circles, and spinal twists can help lubricate the joints, improve mobility, and reduce stiffness and discomfort. Perform these exercises slowly and mindfully, focusing on smooth, controlled movements.

By adapting core exercises for joint health and prioritizing gentle, low-impact movements, seniors can effectively strengthen their core muscles while minimizing the risk of joint pain and discomfort.

Core Workouts for Seniors with Mobility Issues

Mobility issues, such as limited range of motion, balance issues, or difficulty getting up and down from the floor, can present significant challenges when it comes to engaging in core exercises. However, with the right approach and modifications, seniors with mobility issues can still benefit from core workouts. Here are some strategies for adapting core exercises for seniors with mobility issues:

- **Seated Core Exercises:** Many core exercises can be performed while seated in a chair or on a stability ball, making them accessible to seniors with mobility issues. Seated exercises like seated marches, seated torso twists, and seated leg lifts target the core muscles while providing support and stability for those who may have difficulty standing or balancing.

- **Standing Support:** For seniors who are able to stand but may require additional support or assistance, incorporating standing exercises with the use of a chair, wall, or sturdy surface can be beneficial. Standing exercises like standing marches, wall push-ups, and standing side bends can help improve balance, stability, and core strength while providing support for those with mobility issues.

- **Balance and Stability Training:** Balance and stability exercises are essential for seniors with mobility issues, as they help improve proprioception, coordination, and overall stability.

Incorporate balance exercises like single-leg stands, heel-to-toe walks, and balance board exercises into your core workout routine to challenge the core muscles while improving balance and mobility.

- **Modify Traditional Exercises:** Many traditional core exercises can be modified to accommodate seniors with mobility issues. For example, instead of performing traditional planks on the floor, seniors can perform modified planks with support from a wall or elevated surface. Similarly, traditional crunches can be modified by performing them on a stability ball or with the knees bent to reduce strain on the lower back.

- **Use Assistive Devices:** Consider using assistive devices such as resistance bands, stability balls, or foam rollers to provide support and assistance during core exercises. These tools can help seniors with mobility issues perform exercises safely and effectively while reducing the risk of injury.

By incorporating seated core exercises, standing support, balance and stability training, modified traditional exercises, and assistive devices into their core workout routine, seniors with mobility issues can improve core strength, balance, and overall mobility.

Consulting with Healthcare Professionals

Before starting any new exercise program, especially as a senior or individual with existing health concerns, it's essential to consult with healthcare professionals for personalized guidance and support. Healthcare professionals, such as physicians, physical therapists, and certified personal trainers specializing in senior fitness, can provide valuable insight and recommendations tailored to your individual needs and goals. Here are some reasons to consider consulting with healthcare professionals before starting a core workout routine:

- **Assessment of Current Health Status:** Healthcare professionals can assess your current health status, including any existing medical conditions, injuries, or mobility issues that may impact your ability to engage in core exercises safely. They can provide personalized recommendations based on your unique health profile and help you determine the most appropriate exercise program for your needs.

- **Development of a Safe and Effective Exercise Program:** Healthcare professionals can help develop a safe and effective exercise program tailored to your individual needs, goals, and abilities. They can recommend specific core exercises, modifications, and progressions based on your current fitness level, mobility, and any underlying health concerns.

- **Monitoring Progress and Adjusting as Needed:** Healthcare professionals can monitor your progress over time and make adjustments to your exercise program as needed. They can help track your strength, flexibility, balance, and mobility improvements, and modify your workouts accordingly to ensure continued progress and prevent injury or overtraining.

- **Prevention of Injury:** Healthcare professionals can provide guidance on proper form and technique for core exercises to help prevent injury and reduce the risk of exacerbating existing health issues. They can teach you how to perform exercises safely and effectively, and provide feedback and corrections as needed to ensure proper alignment and execution.

- **Motivation and Accountability:** Working with healthcare professionals can provide motivation and accountability to help you stay on track with your core workout routine. They can offer encouragement, support, and guidance along the way, helping you overcome challenges and stay committed to your fitness goals.

Whether it's consulting with your primary care physician for medical clearance, working with a physical therapist for rehabilitation exercises, or seeking guidance from a certified personal trainer for personalized workout programming, consulting with healthcare professionals is an essential step in ensuring safe and effective participation in core exercises, especially for seniors or individuals with mobility issues. special considerations for seniors when it comes to core exercises include adapting exercises for joint health, addressing mobility issues, and consulting with healthcare professionals for personalized guidance and support. By prioritizing gentle, low-impact exercises that minimize stress on the joints, modifying exercises to accommodate mobility issues, and seeking guidance from healthcare professionals, seniors can effectively strengthen their core muscles and improve overall health and well-being. Remember to listen to your body, respect its limits, and prioritize safety and proper technique to ensure a safe and effective workout experience. With the right approach and support, seniors can enjoy the many benefits of a strong and resilient core at any age.

FAQS AND ADDITIONAL RESOURCES

As you embark on your journey to improve core strength and overall fitness, you may have questions and seek additional resources to support your efforts. In this chapter, we'll address common questions, provide recommendations for reading and online resources, and explore ways to find community support to enhance your fitness journey.

Answering Common Questions

Q: What are the benefits of core exercises for seniors?

A: Core exercises offer numerous benefits for seniors, including improved balance, stability, and posture, reduced risk of falls and injuries, enhanced functional mobility for everyday activities, and relief from lower back pain and discomfort. Strengthening the core muscles also supports overall strength and endurance, which can improve overall quality of life and independence as we age.

Q: How often should seniors engage in core exercises?

A: Seniors should aim to engage in core exercises at least two to three times per week, with a day of rest in between sessions to allow for recovery. It's essential to listen to your body and adjust the frequency and intensity of your workouts based on your individual needs and abilities. Starting with shorter, more frequent sessions and gradually increasing duration and intensity over time can help prevent injury and promote steady progress.

Q: Can seniors with existing health conditions or mobility issues still do core exercises?

A: Yes, many core exercises can be modified to accommodate seniors with existing health conditions or mobility issues. It's essential to consult with healthcare professionals, such as physicians or physical therapists, to determine the most appropriate exercises and modifications based on your individual needs and abilities. Seated core exercises, standing support, balance training, and use of assistive devices are all options for seniors with mobility issues.

Q: How long does it take to see results from core exercises?

A: The timeline for seeing results from core exercises can vary depending on individual factors such as current fitness level, consistency with workouts, and adherence to proper nutrition and recovery practices. Generally, most people can expect to start noticing improvements in core strength, stability, and posture within a few weeks to a few months of consistent training. However, it's important to remember that progress may be gradual, and patience and persistence are key to long-term success.

Recommended Reading and Online Resources

For those looking to deepen their understanding of core health and fitness or seeking additional guidance and inspiration, there are numerous books and online resources available. Here are some recommended reading and online resources to support your fitness journey:

1. **"The Complete Idiot's Guide to Core Conditioning" by Dr. Mark Kovacs:** This comprehensive guide provides practical advice, exercises, and strategies for developing a strong and stable core. With clear instructions and illustrations, it's an

excellent resource for beginners and experienced fitness enthusiasts alike.

2. **"Strength Training Anatomy" by Frederic Delavier:** This classic book offers a detailed look at the anatomy of strength training exercises, including those targeting the core muscles. With full-color illustrations and explanations of muscle function and movement, it's a valuable resource for understanding how different exercises engage the core muscles.

3. **Online Resources:**

    *   The American Council on Exercise (ACE): ACE offers a variety of resources, including articles, videos, and workout plans, to help individuals of all ages and fitness levels improve core strength and overall fitness. Their website also features a directory of certified personal trainers and fitness professionals who can provide personalized guidance and support.

    *   National Institute on Aging (NIA): The NIA offers a wealth of resources specifically designed for older adults, including exercise guides, videos, and interactive tools. Their website provides evidence-based information on exercise and physical activity for seniors, with a focus on promoting health, independence, and longevity.

    *   YouTube Channels: There are many YouTube channels dedicated to fitness for seniors, offering free workout videos, tutorials, and tips for improving core strength and overall fitness. Channels such as "Fitness Blender,"

"HASfit," and "Senior Fitness with Meredith" provide a variety of workouts suitable for seniors of all fitness levels.

Finding Community Support

Engaging in core exercises and maintaining a consistent fitness routine can be more enjoyable and motivating with the support of a community. Whether it's connecting with like-minded individuals online or joining local fitness classes or groups, finding community support can help you stay accountable, motivated, and inspired on your fitness journey. Here are some ways to find community support:

- **Online Forums and Social Media Groups:** Joining online forums, Facebook groups, or social media communities focused on fitness for seniors can provide a supportive environment for sharing experiences, asking questions, and finding motivation and inspiration from others on a similar journey. Look for groups that align with your interests and goals and actively participate by sharing your progress and supporting others.

- **Local Fitness Classes and Groups:** Many community centers, senior centers, and fitness facilities offer group exercise classes specifically designed for seniors. Joining a local fitness class or group can provide an opportunity to connect with others in your community, receive personalized instruction and guidance from certified instructors, and enjoy the camaraderie and support of working out with others.

- **Partner Workouts:** Partnering up with a friend, family member, or workout buddy can provide added motivation and accountability for sticking to your fitness routine. Whether it's meeting for regular walks, attending fitness classes together, or sharing workout routines and progress updates, having a workout partner can make exercise more enjoyable and rewarding.

- **Virtual Workouts:** With the rise of virtual fitness platforms and streaming services, it's easier than ever to access live and on-demand workout classes from the comfort of your own home. Joining virtual workout classes or challenges can provide a sense of community and connection with others while allowing you to exercise on your own schedule and at your own pace.

By seeking out community support through online forums, social media groups, local fitness classes, and workout buddies, you can enhance your fitness journey, stay motivated, and enjoy the benefits of improved core strength and overall fitness. this chapter addresses common questions about core exercises for seniors, provides recommendations for reading and online resources to support your fitness journey, and explores ways to find community support for motivation and accountability. Whether you're looking to deepen your knowledge, connect with others, or find inspiration to stay consistent with your workouts, there are plenty of resources and support networks available to help you achieve your core health and fitness goals. Remember to stay curious, keep learning, and reach out for support when needed as you continue on your fitness journey.

CONCLUSION

In this comprehensive guide to core health and fitness for seniors, we've explored the importance of maintaining a strong and resilient core, the benefits of core exercises, and strategies for overcoming common challenges. From understanding the fundamentals of core fitness to addressing special considerations for seniors, each chapter has provided valuable insights and practical tips to help readers improve their core strength, stability, and overall well-being.

Throughout our journey, we've emphasized the importance of listening to your body, respecting its limits, and prioritizing safety and proper technique. Whether you're just starting out on your fitness journey or looking to take your core workouts to the next level, the key is consistency, patience, and persistence. By incorporating core exercises into your routine, making adjustments based on your individual needs and abilities, and seeking support from healthcare professionals and community networks, you can achieve lasting improvements in core health and fitness.

As we conclude this guide, it's important to remember that health is not just about the absence of illness, but rather a state of physical, mental, and emotional well-being. Taking care of your body through regular exercise, proper nutrition, adequate rest, and stress management is essential for maintaining overall health and vitality. As Hippocrates famously said, "Let food be thy medicine and medicine be thy food." This timeless wisdom reminds us of the powerful connection between nutrition and health, and the importance of making informed choices to nourish our bodies and support optimal well-being.

So, as you continue on your journey to improve core health and fitness, remember to approach your goals with curiosity, determination, and a willingness to learn and grow. Celebrate your progress, stay motivated, and don't be afraid to ask for help when needed. With dedication, perseverance, and the right mindset, you can achieve the strong, resilient core you desire and enjoy a life of health, vitality, and active aging.

In the words of Mahatma Gandhi, "It is health that is real wealth and not pieces of gold and silver." As you invest in your health and well-being, you're not only enhancing your quality of life but also building a foundation for a brighter, healthier future. So, keep moving forward, prioritize your health, and remember that every step you take towards better core health is a step towards a happier, more fulfilling life.

As we wrap up our exploration of core exercises and their impact on overall health and fitness, it's clear that there's no one-size-fits-all approach to achieving a strong and resilient core. Throughout this chapter, we've delved into the advantages and disadvantages of 5-minute core exercises, explored strategies for maximizing results, and emphasized the importance of proper form, consistency, and integration into daily life.

From the time-efficiency of 5-minute workouts to the importance of supplementing with full-length sessions, we've learned that variety and balance are key components of a successful core training regimen. By combining short, focused exercises with longer, more comprehensive workouts, individuals can target different muscle groups, stimulate growth and adaptation, and achieve a well-rounded level of fitness.

Moreover, our discussion on proper form and technique underscores the importance of safety and injury prevention in any exercise routine. Whether you're performing a 5-minute plank or a full-length strength training session, prioritizing correct alignment, engagement, and control is essential for maximizing results and minimizing the risk of injury. Remember, quality always trumps quantity when it comes to exercise.

But perhaps the most significant takeaway from our exploration is the idea of integration: integrating core exercises into daily activities, integrating short workouts with longer sessions, and integrating fitness into our overall lifestyle. By making core training a consistent part of our daily routine and incorporating movement into everyday activities, we not only strengthen our core muscles but also improve posture, stability, and overall functional fitness.

As we conclude this chapter, I'm reminded of a quote by the renowned physician and philosopher Maimonides: "The preservation of health is easier than the cure of the disease." These words serve as a powerful reminder that investing in our health and well-being today is the best way to prevent illness and injury in the future. So, let us continue to prioritize our health, make time for exercise, and strive for balance in all aspects of our lives.

To all the readers embarking on their fitness journey, I encourage you to stay committed, stay consistent, and stay curious. Whether you're just starting out or looking to take your core workouts to the next level, remember that every small step forward brings you closer to your goals. Celebrate your progress, learn from setbacks, and never lose sight of the incredible potential that lies within you.

In the end, it's not about achieving perfection or reaching some arbitrary standard of fitness. It's about embracing the journey, enjoying the process, and celebrating the incredible capabilities of the human body. So, keep moving, keep exploring, and above all, keep believing in yourself. Your health and vitality are worth every effort, and with dedication and determination, you can achieve anything you set your mind to.